DURRANI'S

Flash Memory Notes

For

USMLE STEP 3

&

INTERNAL MEDICINE

Examinations

- "Flip Through" at your own pace – ideal for a busy clinician, or for last minute revision.
- Focus on "KEY FACTS" – No Frills High Yield Facts
- Unique Layout – Designed to Boost Visual and Associative recall memory.
- High Yield Facts in a Flip Notes Format to boost your retention of "KEY Clinical Facts", and sharpen your medical test taking skills.

Jameel Durrani, MD FACP FCCP

PREFACE:

These notes are "not" intended to replace standard textbook-based learning of Principals and Practice of Internal Medicine. A thorough basic understanding and familiarity with the core subject matter is an essential pre-requisite.

We have collected precise clinically relevant information from publically available resources, and presented it in a Unique "color-coded and typographically spaced" format designed to reinforce "Visual memorization" and recall of important clinical information, as and when needed.

We have avoided memory clutter by including only the relevant "Take Home" pearls designed to sharpen evidence-based clinical decision making skills.

Medicine is an ever-changing subject. Information presented in this book is solely intended as a memory aid. This information should not be used to cure, diagnose or treat any medical condition or symptoms.

Always consult your physician or designated healthcare provider for any questions regarding any health related matters.

All readers are encouraged to contact us with any comment and suggestions, at jfdurrani@outlook.com

Sincerely,

J. Durrani, MD

CONTENT Layout

1. SIGNS
2. SYMPTOMS
3. SYNDROMES
4. DISEASES
5. THERAPEUTICS
6. OPERATIVE AND PERI-OPERATIVE/TRANSPLANT CARE
7. WOMEN'S HEALTH
8. DIAGNOSTICS
9. INTERPRETATIONS SKILLS

SIGNS:

➢ ATRIAL SEPTAL DEFECT:
FIXED splitting of **S2**.

➢ Physiological splitting of S2:
EXCLUDES aortic stenosis from the differential diagnosis.

➢ TRIGEMINAL NEURALGIA:
- Rx of Choice: CARBAMAZEPINE
- Tricyclic Antidepressants (TCA's) are helpful in other chronic neuropathic pain syndromes.

➤ WADDELL'S SIGN:
- To assess **non organic (Fictitious) Back Pain**.
- Pain on Axial Load testing, but discordant results on straight leg raising, while sitting and Supine.
- Rx: Psychological Eval and Cognitive Behavioral Therapy (CBT)

➤ TINNEL'S TEST:
- Tapping the Posterior Tibial nerve behind the Medial Malleolus elicits Pain – Diagnostic for **TARSAL TUNNEL SYNDROME**

➤ SPURLING's Maneuver:
- Used to Diagnose **CERVICAL RADICULOPATHY**
- **Arm Pain elicited by Neck Flexion TOWARDS the affected side.**
- Treatment: NSAIDS + Moist Heat +/- Soft Collar

SYMPTOMS

➢ **UNEXPLAINED FEVER in patients with PROSTHETIC VALVES:**

    Always Consider risk of **Bacterial infection/valve abscess** <<<

    Diagnostic test of choice: **TEE**

➢ **SUDDEN SYNCOPE IN A CHF PATIENT:**

    <u>Ominous sign</u> in systolic heart failure.

    High risk for sudden death.

    <u>**Assess FOR AICD PLACEMENT**</u>.

➢ **BUTTOCK PAIN**

D/D: **SPINAL STENOSIS:**

      Pain increases with standing and walking

      Improved on BENDING FORWARD or SITTING

  LEG ISCHEMIA:

      Worse with activity

      >20% drop in ABI with exercise

ATYPICAL CHEST PAIN WORKUP:

>>>> ALGORITHMS:

ANGIOGRAPHY: **HIGH risk factors**: (+ MI profile, low BP, EKG changes, LV Dysfx .)

EXERCISE STRESS TEST: Atypical pain + **normal EKG**.

EXERCISE PERFUSION IMAGING: Atypical pain + **abnormal EKG** and **no high risk factors**.

PATIENTS WITH CHEST PAIN AT REST (abnormal EKG, elevated cardiac enzymes):

>>> **Stress Echo is CONTRAINDICATED**.

Early invasive approach is recommended.

ACUTE DYSPNEA in a POST-MI:

Rule out:

Papillary muscle rupture

Ventricular septal defect.

➤ ACUTE MITRAL REGURGITATION (MR) AFTER MI

MR due to papillary muscle rupture after MI often **improves after coronary revascularization**.

➤ HEARTBURN:

- Dyspepsia without Alarm Features (Anemia, weight loss, Vomiting) can be empirically treated for H. Pylori infection. (Serologic test and Treat) approach.

➤ MENIERE'S DISEASE:

- **Most Common cause** of Disabling Vertigo
- Usual Age of onset: 4th to 6th decade of life.
- May lead to progressive low frequency sensorineural hearing loss.
- D/D: Benign Positional Vertigo (BPV) and Vestibular Neuronitis, Vestibular Labyrinthitis

- **BENIGN POSITIONAL VERTIGO (BPV):**
  - **BRIEF Episodes of vertigo (<1 min), starting with CHANGE in HEAD POSITION**
  - 1st Rx option:
    - Habituation Exercises
    - Canalolith repositioning (EPLEY's Maneuver)
  - 2nd Rx Option:
    - Meclizine for severe intractable symptoms, ie, Labyrinthitis, Meniere's disease.

- **VESTIBULAR NEURONITIS:**
  - Single Episode of Disabling Vertigo, +/- Dizziness, that may LAST FEW DAYS

- **VESTIBULAR LABYRINTHITIS:**
  - Same as Vestibular Neuronitis, PLUS UNILATERAL HEARING LOSS

- **ACUTE HEARING LOSS in ONE EAR and NORMAL EXAM:**
  - **Systemic Corticosteroids** have been found to be helpful, if given **promptly**, alongwith **an ENT Referral.**

- **EPSITAXIS:**
  - Bleeding is considered ANTERIOR Epistaxis if no airway management needed, and stable hemodynamics status.
  - POSTERIOR Epsitaxis requires ENT consultation and may need airway management.

- **DYSFUNCTIONAL UTERINE BLEEDING (DUB):**
  - GLOD Standard for Diagnostic Workup:
    - ENDOMETRIAL BIOPSY

- **URINARY INCONTINENCE:**
  - **NORTRYPTYLLINE** – can WORSEN Incontinence..
  - **ESTROGEN Therapy**: can also WORSEN incontinence.

- **URGE INCONTINENCE:**
  - TOLTERODINE is preferred over OXYBUTININ
  - Fewer CNS Side effects, and Less dry mouth.

- **Joint Pain in Injection drug abuse patient:**
  - HIGH RISK for MRSA and Pseudomonas Arthritis

➢ JOINT Pain in A PROSTHETIC JOINT
- ALWAYS ASPIRATE AND CULTURE the Joint Fluid.

➢ TRAVELLER'S DIARRHEA:

Most COMMON causes
- DEVELOPING COUNTRIES:
  - E.COLI (Entero-toxigenic)
- USA
  - CAMPYLOBACTER JEJUNI
  - Risk Factors:
    - Poultry
    - Cross contaminated utensils and counter-tops

➢ WATERY SPUTUM
- (with High Fever, Hemoptysis, Sepsis)
- Dx: **PNEUMONIC PLAGUE**
- Rx: **IV STREPTOMYCINE**
- 100% Mortality if not treated with Streptomycin in time.

- **CHRONIC DIGITAL ULCER/NODULE**
    - Rule out **MYCOBACTERIUM MARINUM INFECTION** by **BIOPSY and Histopath Exam**
    - Rx: **Macrolides, Sulfonamides, Rifampin Ethambutol.**
    - **M.Marinum is RESISTANT TO INH, PAS & STREPTOMYCINE**

- **4 D's of BOTULISM:**
    - **Dysphagia**
    - **Dysarthria**
    - **Dysphonia**
    - **Diplopia**

- **MIGRAINE:**
    - Attacks can transform into **CHRONIC DAILY HEADACHES** with frequent use (>3/week) use of NSAIDS, tryptans and Butalbitol.

- **SUDDEN SEVERE HEADACHE:**
    - "RED FLAG SIGNS" (That requires immediate Neuro/Radiology eval:
        - ACUTE onset in Patients MORE THAN 50 Years of age.
        - Positive HIV status, Non-resolving neuro deficits, Fever, Rash, Vomiting, Severe HTN.
        - Severe Headache following ANY Trauma.

- **Age Related Benign FORGETFULLNESS:**
    - Does NOT increase risk of Alzheimer's Disease
    - Workup to rule out Vitamin B12, Folate Deficiency, Rapid Plasma Reagent (RPPR) testing for Syphilis. CBC may be normal early in EARLY B12 Deficiency.

- ➢ **SHOULDER PAIN- DIFFERENTIAL DIAGNOSIS:**
    - **Rotator Cuff Tendonitis**
        - **Pain on Mid-Arc Abduction** is Diagnostic
    - **Rotator Cuff Tear:**
        - Inability to <u>SMOOTHLY</u> bring down the abducted arm to the side, is a SPECIFIC diagnostic test (but not very SENSITIVE)

- ➢ **KNEE PAIN WITH "POPPING" SENSATION**
    - Due to Meniscal tear
    - Pain worse going up and down stairs
    - RX:
        - Knee strengthening exercises.
        - Avoid Stair Stepper

- ➢ **HEEL PAIN:**
    - Most common Cause: **PLANTAR FASCITIS**
    - **TINNEL'S TEST:**

Tapping the posterior tibial nerve behind the Medial Malleolus elicits Pain – Diagnostic for **TARSAL TUNNEL SYNDROME.**

➤ DRY EYES:

(Refractory to Moisture Replacement Therapy):
- **1st Rx Option: CEVIMELINE**: A cholinergic agent with muscarinic Agonist properties at M1 and M3 Receptors found in exocrine glands.
- **2nd Rx option: Pilocarpine**, Although it can cause Excessive sweating.

➤ THICK DYSTRPOHIC (UGLY) NAILS:

- Diagnostic test of choice: **Proximal Nail bed Debris Culture** to confirm/rule out Fungal nail infection (Onychomycosis)
- D/D: Psoriasis can have similar appearance.

➤ SYNCOPE:

- **SITUATIONAL SYNCOPE:**
  - AKA "**Vasovagal Syncope**"
  - In situations with Excessive Vagal Stimulation.
- **CAROTID SINUS SYNCOPE**
  - Strictly due to pressure on the Carotid Sinus, i.e, Head turning, tight Collar, or a tumor in the carotid sinus area.

CHANGES IN VISION:

- **DRY MACULAR DEGENERATION**
  - Symptoms: Faded colors, may be unilateral.
  - Age Related process
  - Retinal "**DRUZENS**", areas of loss of epithelial pigment on the Retina.

- **WET MACULAR DEGENERATION:**
  - **Neovascularization** process in Choroid.

- **CATARACT:**
  - **Lens opacification** on Eye Exam
  - Decreased visual Acuity
    - D/D: **IMMATURE** Nuclear Cataract
      - Red Reflex with central Opacity
      - **PRESERVED Vision**

- **DIABETIC PROLIFERATIVE RETINOPATHY:**
  - "Cotton-Wool" Spots on Retina
  - Retinal Micro aneurysm
  - NEW and Dilated Retinal Vessels

- **VITREOUS HEMORRHAGE:**
  - **Eye is Neither RED nor PAINFUL**
  - Retinal details are obscured on Ophthalmoscopy

SYNDROMES

➤ MARFAN SYNDROME:

High risk for Aortic root Dilatation

Associated with Aortic regurgitation

>>> Study of choice: **2-D echo**

>>> Elective **aortic root replacement:** when diameter >5 cm.

➤ NOONAN syndrome:

Pulmonic valve stenosis.

➤ WPW (Wolff-Parkinson-White syndrome)

A type of **AV reentrant tachycardia** <<<

Short PR with Delta waves

>>> AVOID AV Nodal blocking drugs i.e., **METOPROLOL and VERAPAMIL**, as these drugs can increase conduction through the accessory pathway.

- ➢ **NEUROLEPTIC MALIGNANT SYNDROME (NMS):**
  - o Distinguishing feature from other hyperthermic states (i.e, Thyroid Storm, Malignant Hyperthermia) is **RIGIDITY.**

- ➢ **Irritable Bowel Syndrome (IBS)**
  - o **Diarrhea Predominant Type:**
    - **LOPERAMIDE**
      - Established 1st Line Therapy.
    - **ALOSETRON:**
      - FDA approved for Resistant cases of Diarrhea predominant IBS.
      - Use with caution as it can cause Ischemic Colitis in a small number of patients.
  - o **Fiber is Not Better than Placebo** in IBS.

- **PROPOFOL INFUSION SYNDROME:**
  - RARE
  - Seen in ICU patients on Propofol infusion, alongwith vasopressors and steroids therapies.
  - Highest risk **seen with higher dosage (>75mcg/Kg/min), and duration (>48 Hrs)**
  - Propofol can impair free fatty acids metabolism, and impair mitochondrial activity
  - **Features:**
    - Severe Metabolic Acidosis
    - Cardiac Failure
    - Rhabdomyolysis
    - Renal Failure and Hyperkalemia

- **HEREDITARY HEMORRHAGIC TELENGIECTASIA**
  - Arteriovenous Malformation (AVM) and Pulmonary Hypertension
  - Mutation on **Chromosome 12 q 13**
  - **FINDINGS:**
    - Epistaxis
    - Telengiectasias: on Fingers, nose, lips, and oral cavity.
    - Visceral AVM lesions in GI and Resp Tract.
    - 1st Degree relatives with similar conditions

- **SILICOSIS:**
  - Also seen in SURFACE MINING workers.
  - Apical Nodular Opacities on CXR, may coalesce to make large mass-like lesions, called "PROGRESSIVE MASSIVE FIBROSIS (PMF)
  - PMF patients at high risk for TB.

- **TOXIC SHOCK SYNDROME:**
  - Can be from Staph or Streptococcal infection
  - Rx of Choice: VANCOMYCIN + CLINDAMYCIN

- **METABOLIC SYNDROME:**
  - Any THREE of the following:
    - Increased Waist Circumference
    - High Triglycerides
    - LOW HDL
    - HYPERTENSION
    - High Fasting Blood Glucose
  - Rx: Intensive Lifestyle modification

- **CHURG STRAUSS SYNDROME:**
  - Asthma with SMALL VESSELL VASCULITIS, pulmonary infiltrates, eosinophilia in the setting of Starting A NEW Leukotriene Receptor Antagonist (LTRA), AND WITHDRAWL of steroids.

DISEASES

➢ CARDIOGENIC SHOCK:

Peripheral hypoperfusion with **cool extremities**:

>>> may exist without mental status changes.

Consider adding inotropic support, i.e. **Milrinone**

➢ STEMI with HYPERTENSION:

(uncontrolled i.e, BP more than 180/110):

PROCEED WITH PCI (revascularization), preferred choice has thrombolytics are relatively contraindicated.

➢ DIASTOLIC HEART FAILURE:

"<u>CHF with NORMAL EF</u>".

<u>**SPIRONOLACTONE is NOT helpful**</u>. No proven benefit in diastolic heart failure.

<u>**ARBs may reduce hospitalization**</u> but no impact on mortality.

➤ DECOMPENSATED HEART FAILURE:

Biventricular pacer is indicated. (NYHA 3 and 4).

Biventricular pacer is also indicated for QTc > 120 msec

➤ ATRIAL SEPTAL DEFECTS (ASD):

Mid septal defects (**SECUNDUM** type): No valvular involvement. **Treated by PERCUTANEOUS DEVICE closure**.

Lower septal defects (**PRIMUM** type): **+ CLEFT in Mitral or Tricuspid valve. Treated by SURGICAL CLOSURE**.

Early closure it is recommended in asymptomatic patients with evidence of volume overload.

➤ REPAIRED TETRALOGY OF FALLOT:

Most common long-term complication is **PULMONARY VALVE REGURGITATION**.

Other complications include: Late onset A. fib, and VSD (Holosystolic murmur, **not changing with respiration**).

➤ MYOCARDITIS:

Recommended Rx: **Supportive care for Heart failure**

NO ROLE for NSAIDs and steroids.

Ace inhibitors are recommended.

>>> Troponins may be elevated.

➤ CYANOTIC HEART DISEASE:

Normal hemoglobin in these patients: **18-21 Gm** <<<

High risk for **relative Iron deficiency** (hemoglobin less than **18 g**) due to recurrent phlebotomies.

TREATMENT: Iron therapy for 7-10 days.

SYMPTOMS: Dyspnea and fatigue

➤ SUSTAINED SYMPTOMATIC SVT:

AICD placement improves survival.

- **ALCOHOLIC CARDIOMYOPATHY**

    A form of : **DILATED CARDIOMYOPATHY <<<**

- **INFERIOR WALL MI (ST ELEVATION IN LEAD II, III and AVF) with CARDIOGENIC SHOCK:**

    = **RV infarct <<<**

    Treatment includes **volume challenge with saline,**

    >>> **Prefer volume challenge over IABP.**

- **AORTIC STENOSIS - with symptoms (CHF etc.)**

    TREATMENT OF CHOICE: **AVR**

    Valvuloplasty and percutaneous treatment options have not shown outcome benefit. **AVR is preferred.**

    Ace inhibitors are relatively contraindicated in significant aortic stenosis.

    Symptoms in **worsening AORTIC STENOSIS may be insidious** i.e. "exertional dyspnea ", but **still warrant valve replacement** recommendation.

➤ COARCTATION OF AORTA

BICUSPID VALVE STATUS is common.

Radiofemoral delay is noted.

➤ AORTIC DISSECTION:

Acute aortic dissection can have **associated ischemia in RCA territory** (lead 2, 3 and aVF changes).

➤ AORTIC TRANSECTION:

Always a concern with history of trauma, which may be a remote event.

Physical examination may be "normal" entirely.

➤ AORTIC VALVE SCLEROSIS:

Carries **INCREASED RISK of cardiovascular events**, up to 50%.

Evaluate for other cardiac risk factors, EVEN in asymptomatic patients (lipid profile, etc.) with aortic valve sclerosis.

➤ BICUSPID aortic valve with AORTIC REGURGITATION:

Long-term **Nifedipine** in **asymptomatic** patients + serial ECHO.

AVReplacement (AVR) for **symptomatic** patients, EF less than 60%, LV end-systolic diameter more than 55 mm.

➤ MITRAL REGURGITATION:

Holosystolic murmur **MAX at apex**.

Radiates to axilla.

No respiratory variation.

➤ RADIATION-INDUCED RESTRICTIVE CARDIOMYOPATHY:

NORMAL LV THICKNESS on echo with restrictive filling and no respiratory variation.

D/D

CHEMOTHERAPY-INDUCED CARDIOMYOPATHY:

shows VENTRICULAR DILATATION and impaired systolic function on echo.

➤ VIRAL PERICARDITIS:

Can cause subacute pericardial tamponade without constriction.

Treat with pericardiocentesis.

Pericardiectomy is only indicated for constrictive pericarditis.

➤ AV nodal reentrant tachycardia (AVNRT):

Narrow complex tachycardia + No visible P WAVES.

D/D   (P waves are VISIBLE in AVR T)

First treatment for atrial tachycardia-carotid sinus massage

NEXT STEP: ADENOSINE -treatment of choice for narrow complex SVT.

➤ HOCM murmur:

INCREASES with VALSALVA maneuver

DECREASES with HANDGRIP and PASSIVE LEG RAISING.

➤ Premature ventricular contractions (PVCs):

Rate control or heart rate suppression is **only recommended with SEVERE AND DISABLING symptoms**.

➤ CARDIAC TUMORS:

Rare

\>>> **Can cause fever, weight loss, increased ESR and anemia.**

➤ CROHN'S DISEASE:
- **SKIP Lesions**, and **RECTAL Sparing**
- Deep Ulcers, with risk for fistula formation
- Higher incidence in smokers
- D/D: Ulcerative Colitis; UC has continuous lesions and usually involves the Rectum. Incidence of UC is more in former or non smokers.

➤ ACUTE GALLSTONE PANCREATITIS:
- After initial pain control and rehydration, FIRST Diagnostic test of choice **is ABDOMINAL Ultrasound (not ERCP).**
- ERCP is only indicated when if ductal dilatation is noted on Ultrasound, +/- jaundice develops with significant worsening of LFTs.

- **Hypoventilation due to Neuro Muscular Disease (NMD)**
    - Rx of choice is Noninvasive Ventilation (NIV)
    - NMD causes a RESTRICTIVE pattern on pulmonary Function Testing.
    - **20-30-40 Rule:** to decide need for intubation
        - Vital Capacity < 20 ml/Kg
        - Max Insp Pressure (MIP) < 30 cm H2O
        - Max Exp Pressure (MEP) <40 cm H2O
        - & inability to maintain secretions

- **HYPERTENSIVE EMERGENCY:**
    - Goal is to reduce MAP by 20-25%
    - Sodium Nitroprusside (NIPRIDE) is an arterial and Venodilator. It can be rapidly Titrated.
    - Add LABETOLOL (for Rate Control) in patients with risk of aortic Dissection.

- **Rheumatoid Arthritis (RA) related Lung Disease (ILD):**
    - Trigger Can Be either
        - **DISEASE RELATED** effect, or
        - **DRUG RELATED** Effect (i.e, Methotrexate) , or
        - **Opportunistic pulmonary Infections** secondary to immunocompromised status FROM ra DRUGS, i.e, TNF-Alpha
    - Look for **Time relationships**, i.e, start of new medications and worsening of Lung symptoms.

- **ASTHMA –Diagnosis and Management**
  - **Recurrent Asthma Episodes in young patients :**
    - **Laryngoscopy** is recommended to rule out Vocal Cord Dysfunction **(VCD).**
    - **"ADDUCTION"** noted during **INSPIRATION**, confirms the diagnosis of VCD.
  - **Loss of Asthma Control** (in previously well controlled Asthmatics):
    - Consider a short course of oral corticosteroids.
  - **Persistent Asthma**:
    - Start with Inhaled Corticosteroid AND Short Acting Beta Agonist (ICS + SABA)
  - **Severe Asthma Exacerbations:**
    - Primary Rx: **SABA +Anticholinergic Nebs**
    - **HELIOX and NPPV** are not proven as PRIMARY Therapies
  - **Reactive Airway Dysfunction Syndrome (RADS)**
    - Follows **SINGLE LARGE exposures** (fumes/Spills/Vapors) to agents that can damage airways.

- ➢ **ASTHMA – (Cont'd.)**
  - **A positive Methacholine Challenge Test** is needed to confirm the Diagnosis.
  - o **Positive Methacholine Challenge test without Symptoms**
    - No Rx is recommended without symptoms.

- ➢ **COPD**
  - o **Inhaled corticosteroids Do NOT change the rate of decline in FEV1.**
  - o Patients with **GOLD COPD Stage 4 (FEV1 < 30% of predicted, of < 50% or predicted with presence of chronic Respiratory failure on Oxygen therapy)** presenting with exacerbations, should be treated as Community acquired Pneumonia

- ➢ **CORPULMONALE:**
  - o Pulmonary HTN secondary to a (primary) Lung Disease, i.e, COPD
  - o Usually occurs in GOLD COPD Stage 3 & 4.
  - o Unlikely if FEV1 > 1L
  - o If Pulm HTN is noted with FEV1 > 1L, look for other causes, i.e, OSAS, OHS.

- **Cystic Fibrosis with PNEUMOTHORAX**
    - Rx of 1st Choice: **Tube Thoracostomy**
    - Follow with interventions to prevent Recurrence.

- **ACNE:**
    - **Oral Retin-A** is only FDA Approved for Nodular Recalcitrant Acne Only.
    - **FIRST RX Option:**
        - Oral Antibiotics and Topical Antibiotic cream

- **Comedonal Acne**

    (Black and White Heads)
    - **Topical Retinoid** is indicated
    - No relationship between Fast Foods, Chocolate and incidence of Acne.

- ## WEST NILE VIRUS infection:
  - Most common in ELDERLY >65 YEARS OLD
  - Can be transmitted by Blood transfusion (if donor was in asymptomatic period.)
  - Marked WEAKNESS (LMN type) & severe HEADACHE.

- ## ROCKY MOUNTAIN SPOTTED FEVER:
  - **ENTEROVIRAL** illness
  - Sx: Fever, RASH on extremities (UE and LE)
    - **Rash includes PALMS and SOLES**
  - Rx: URGENT **DOXYCYCLINE**

- ## DENGUE FEVER:
  - Severe Headache, Fever, Arthralgia
  - Leukopenia, Thrombocytopenia
  - Dengue Hemorrhagic fevere has capillary fragility and Petechial Rash

- ➢ **NORO VIRUS** infection:
  - ○ **Diarrheal** disease

- ➢ **ADENOVIRUS infection:**
  - ○ Causes CNS Symptoms

- ➢ **POLYOMA JC Virus:**
  - ○ Causes Progressive Multifocal Leukoencephalopathy **(PML)**

- ➢ **POLYOMA BK VIRUS:**
  - ○ DOES NOT cause CNS DISEASE
  - ○ Causes **NEPHROPATHY** and Deteriorating Renal Function (BK = Bad Kidneys).

- **SMALL POX:**
  - **SAME-STAGE** Rash
  - Most on **FACE** and **EXTREMITIES**
  - Incubation period: 7-14 days
  - Contact Isolation protocol: Check their Temperature Q 12 hrs. ISOLATE ALL that develop temp More than 38F/101F

- **VIRAL HEMORRHAGIC FEVER:**
  - 10 Different RNA Viruses
  - MARBURG Virus MOST Deadly
  - POTENTIAL BIOCHEMICAL WEAPONS:
    - MARBURG
    - EBOLA
    - LASSA
  - SYMPTOMS: Fever, Headache, Myalgia, Vomiting and Diarrhea
  - Other names: Argentine/Bolivian Hemorrhagic Fever.

- **AFRICAN TICK BITE FEVER:**
  - **Most Common Rickettsia infection in the world**

- **INFLUENZA/H1N1/H5N1:**
  - Viral Prodrome followed by Bilateral pneumonia and Acute Respiratory Failure.
  - **AMANTADINE**: needs Dose adjustment in Renal patients
  - **RIMANTIDINE**: Rapid Resistance can develop.
  - **OSELTAMIVIR** Side Effect: Metallic Taste.
  - No renal dose adjustment is needed for Oseltamivir and Zanamivir.

- **PULMONARY ASPERGILLOSIS**
  - ACUTE ANGLE BRANCHING on HistoPath Slide
  - IMMUNOCOMPROMISED HOST
  - DIFLUCAN "DOES NOT" TREAT ASPERGILLUS.
  - RX: VORICONAZOLE
  - PSEUDOALLECHERIA :
    - looks just like Aspergillus, on slide, d/d only by Fungal Culture.
    - Rx: Voriconazole (Amphotericin is not effective against PseudoAllecheria)

- **CYCLOSPORA INFECTION**
  - Copious Diarrhea in **International Travelers**
  - **POSITIVE AFB STAIN** on Stool sample
  - **NO FEVER**

- ➢ **E.COLI (Entero-Toxigenic) INFECTION:**
  - Can cause HEMOLYTIC UREMIC SYNDROME (HUS) – due to SHIGA TOXIN.
  - HUS can lead to RENAL FAILURE.

- ➢ **STAPH AUREUS INFECTIONS (INVASIVE types)**
  - 50% may not respond to vancomycin despite IN-VITRO SENSITIVITY.
  - SWITCH Treatment to DAPTOMYCINE.

- ➢ **COMMUNITY ACQUIRED PNEUMONIA (CAP):**
  - CURB-65: Level of care score
  - Rx of 1ST CHOICE: Ceftriaxone + Azithromycin
  - Avoid Levaquin as FIRST choice due to emergence of resistance to intestinal flora.
  - OUTPATIENT Rx of UNCOMPLICATED CAP
    - Macrolides
    - ketolides
    - Doxycycline

- ➤ **ANAEROBIC ASPIRATION PNEUMONIA**
  - RX: CLINDAMYCINE
  - Flagyl does not cover microaerophilic and aerobic streptococci from oral flora.

- ➤ **LEGIONELLA PNEUMONIA:**
  - Peak time are **Late Summer** and **Early Fall**

- ➤ **NOSOCOMIAL DIARRHEA:**
  - Most common causes:
    - Clostridium Difficile (Spores)
    - Norovirus (virions)
  - STRICT Handwashing, STRICT cleaning of all Patient Care areas and CONTACT Isolation
  - Environmental Cultures: NOT Recommended.

- **DISSEMINATED GONOCOCCAL INFECTION:**
  - "DERMATITIS-ARTHRITIS SYNDROME"
  - Pustular skin lesions and asymmetric Joint pains
  - DX: Cultures from Pharynx, Anus and Cervix

- **EPIDIDIMYTIS in a sexually active young male**
  - Can be related to Anal-receptive intercourse
  - Rx Choice #1: Doxycycline + Ceftriaxone, to cover chlamydia and Neisseria Gonorrhea respectively.
  - Rx Choice #2: Fluoroquinolone monotherpay is OK in where enteric organisms are likely, and in patients more than 35 years old.

- **NON-GONOCOCCAL SEPTIC ARTHRITIS:**
  - Staph and Streptococcal infections are most common causes.
  - Rheumatoid Arthritis patients who develop Septic Arthritis:
    - \> 90% have Staph Aureus Infection.

- **Crutzfeld-Jacob Disease (CJD):**
  - Dementia, Dystonia, Behaviour and Personality Changes.
  - 90% Patients die within ONE YEAR.

- **LISTERIA MENINGITIS**
  - Rx options:
    - AMPICILLIN, or
    - Penicillin(PCN)-G + Aminoglycoside
  - PCN Allergic Patients:
    - Bactrim

- **BABESIOSIS:**
  - Tick Born
  - NO SYMPTOMS in Immune Competent Patients
  - SEVERE Symptoms in Immune compromised Patients
  - RX:
    - ATOVAQUONE + ZITHROMAX for symptomatic patients.

- ➤ **EHRLICHIOSIS:**
  - o New name is Human Granulocytic Anaplasmosis
  - o Blood Smear shows "MORULAE" (Ehrlichia inclusion bodies within WBC's.
  - o Rx: Doxycycline

- ➤ **LICHEN SIMPLEX:**
  - o "SCRATCH", that "ITCHES"
  - o A Form of chronic dermatitis where the skin inflammation causes the skin to get scaly and itchy.

- ➤ **ANOREXIA NERVOSA with Hypokalemia**

  (even borderline Hypokalemia):
  - o **ADMIT patient for INPATIENT therapy** due to high risk of severe electrolyte disturbance following Refeeding.

- ➢ **VARICOSE VEINS TREATMENT:**
  - LASER Rx is NOT RECOMMENDED
  - Equal Recommendations for Surgery (Vein Stripping) and SCLEROTHERAPY.

- ➢ **VENOUS ULCERS- Local Rx options:**
  - Hydrocolloid occlusive dressing helps with healing
  - ASPIRIN: (Dose MORE THAN 300 mg Dailiy.

- ➢ **REFLEX SYMPATHETEIC DYSTROPHY (RSD):**
  - AKA: **Complex Regional Pain Syndrome (CRPS)**
  - Follows Limb injury/Vascular event
  - Symptoms: Pain, Paresthesia, vasomotor instability, and PATCHY bone demineralization
  - RX: Analgesics and **BISPHOSPHONATES**.

- **URTICARIAL VASCULITIS:**
  - Skin Biopsy is recommended if no response to antihistamine Rx
  - Presence of LEUKOCYTOCLASTIC VASCULITIS, confirms diagnosis
  - **Differential Diagnosis:**
    - **C-1 Estrase inhibitor Deficiency:**
      - AKA HEREDITARY ANGIOEDEMA
      - Occurs in Women
      - Diagnosed by Low levels of CH50 and C4 during the Attack.

- **OSTEOARTHRITIS and Weight Management:**
  - **No documented improvement in OA with weight Loss alone.**
  - Weight management does help with:
    - BP Management
    - Improved Lipid Profile
    - Reduces progression of Type 2 Diabetes Mellitus.

- **FIBROMYALGIA :**
  - Graded Exercise Therapy is Helpful
  - Massage is not proven to be helpful.

- **CELIAC SPRUE:**
  - May have NO GI distress/diarrhea
  - OSteomalacia and Osteoporosis are common due to malabsorption.

- **CONJUNCTIVITIS:**
  - **VIRAL Conjunctivitis:**
    - PAINLESS RED EYE
    - Clear Discharge
    - No change in visual Acuity
    - Antihistamines and Topical Antibiotics are not Indicated.
  - **BACTERIAL Conjunctivitis:**
    - Purulent Ocular Discharge
  - **Allergic Conjunctivitis:**
    - Red Eye with PRURITIS/ITCHING and Bilateral Symptoms.
    - Rx with Antihistamines.

- **Fulminant Keratitis in patient with Contact Lens**
  - High Risk for PSEUDOMONAS Fulminant Keratitis.
  - Higher risk in Extended wear type Soft Contact Lenses.

- **Ventricular Fibrillation:**
  - ACLS Management Protocol
    - Defibrillation AND
    - **COTE**:
      - **C**PR +
      - **O**xygen +
      - **T**ubes (IV and ETT) +
      - **E**pinephrine /Vasopressin.

THERAPEUTICS

Anti-Arrhythmic Drug Therapy:

- **Class-I**
  - **Na$^+$ Channel Blockers**
    - **Procainamide (Pronestyl):**
      - 15mg/Kg Loading dose, 1-6 mg/min IV continuous dose.
      - Avoid in Severe LV Dysfunction
    - **Flecainide (Tambocor):**
      - 2mg/Kg IV for chemical cardioversion
      - 50-150 mg PO Q 12 maintenance dose.

- **Class-II**
  - **β-Blockers (Sympatholytics)**
    - **Metoprolol:**
      - 5mg Q 5 min IV route, or 50-100 mg PO Q 12 hrs
    - **Esmolol**
      - 0.05 - 0.2 mg/Kg/min infusion
    - **Atenolol**
      - 5mg Q 5 min IV route, or 25-100 mg PO Daily

- Does not Cross Blood Brain Barrier

- **Class-III**
  - **K⁺ Channel Blockers**
    - **Amiodarone**
      - MultiChannel Blocker (Na⁺,K⁺ Blocker)
      - IV Loading Regimen: 150 - 300 mg IV Bolus in D5W, followed by 1mg/min x 6 Hrs, and then 0.5 mg/min x 12 Hrs
      - PO: 400 – 800 mg PO daily in divided doses
    - **Sotalol (Betapace):**
      - β – Blockers, and K⁺ Channel Blocker
      - 80-240 mg PO Q 12 Hrs

- **Class-IV**
  - **Ca⁺⁺ Channel Blockers**
    - **Cardizem:**
      - IV : 0.2 – 0.3 mg/Kg IV Bolus, followed by 5 – 15 mg/Hr Maintenance dose.

- PO: 120 – 360 mg PO daily as sustained release (SR).

- **Class-V**
  - **Digoxin:**
    - Na^+/K^+ - Pump Inhibitor
    - 0.75 – 1.5 mg PO/IV in 3-4 divided doses over 24 hours, then 0.125 – 0.5 mg IV/PO Daily.

  - **Adenosine:**
    - Direct NODE Inhibitor:
    - 6mg followed by 12 mg, may repeat 12 mg againx1.

  - **Magnesium Sulphate:**
    - 2 Gm IV for Torsades De Pointes.

➤ INOTROPIC DRUGS DOSING:

DOPAMINE =

    3-5 µg/kg/minute (**RENAL DOSE**)

    5-10 µg/Kg/minute (vasodilator/inotropic dose)

    >10 µg/Kg/minute (**vasoconstrictor** dose)

DOBUTAMINE:

    5-20 µg/Kg/minute (inotropic >vasodilator)

MILRINONE:

    0.25 - 0.75 µg/Kg/minute (vasodilator >inotropic)

    (+/- 25-50 µg/Kg BOLUS)

➤ PRESSORS WITH DOSING:

EPINEPHRINE:

    1-20 mcg/min = inotropic/vasodilator

    >20 mcg/min = vasoconstrictor

NOREPINEPHRINE (LEVOPHED):

    1-2 mcg/min: Inotropic

>2 mcg/m: Vasoconstrictor

PHENYLEPHRINE (NEO-SYNEPHRINE):

Inotropic: 0.1-0.5 µg/Kg/min

Shock treatment: 40-60 mcg/min (may start at 100-180 mcg/min)

VASOPRESSIN: 0.01 - 0.04 U/min

➢ **Pradaxa (DABIGATRAN):**

Direct Thrombin inhibitor Anticoagulant

Approved for **Non-valvular A. fib anticoagulation**.

Dose = 150 mg by mouth every 12 hours.

➢ NYHA CLASS II PATIENTS WITH PRIOR MI HISTORY:

>>> **AICD** has been show to **add survival benefit**, as a primary prevention against ventricular arrhythmias.

Addition of **spironolactone** is recommended for NYHA **class III and class IV**.

➢ OUT OF HOSPITAL CARDIAC ARREST:

"TIME TO DEFIBRILLATION" is the MOST IMPORTANT DETERMINANT of survival.

Even more important than "TIME TO CPR".

➢ POST-MI CARE PLAN:

ADD STATIN:

REGARDLESS of cholesterol level.

Shown to reduce late cardiovascular events.

➢ NSTEMI/unstable angina:

GPIIB-IIIa inhibitors are indicated.

➢ ACUTE VIRAL PERICARDITIS TREATMENT:

Always add Indomethacin OR other high-dose NSAIDs.

➢ USE OF BETA BLOCKERS IN HEART FAILURE:

Recommended due to improved outcomes.

Titrate dosage according to heart rate effect.

➤ BLACK PATIENTS with CONGESTIVE HEART FAILURE (who are symptomatic on maximized medical therapy):

Consider adding **HYDRALAZINE and NITRATES**.

HYDRALAZINE reduce Afterload and indirectly increase cardiac output. Mortality benefit was also noted.

➤ DIGOXIN TOXICITY:

Fatigue/nausea/anorexia

Atrial tachycardia can occur with variable block

➤ WIDE-COMPLEX TACHYCARDIA (unclear Etiology):

>>> Rx of CHOICE:

PROCAINAMIDE: #1

IBUTILIDE: #2

>>> **Avoid Adenosine** in Atrioventricular Rentrant Tachycardia (AVRT) with pre-excitation, as it carries 2-5% risk of inducing VFib and hemodynamic collapse.

"Pre-Op Heparin Bridge-over" Protocol for Patients with Mechanical Valve, who are on Warfarin Anticoagulation:

MITRAL VALVE:

ALWAYS Bridge with HEPARIN ~ 3 days

AORTIC VALVE:

LOW RISK: OK to stop Coumadin for 3-4 days prior to surgery.

CHRONIC ATRIAL FIBRILLATION:

Decision to Anticoagulate is based on :

CHAD S-2 score: CAD, HTN, Age >75, DM, Stroke/TIA

Conversion to sinus rhythm has **NOT been shown to improve survival**.

ASA (aspirin) is enough for prophylaxis in patients with no risk factors for stroke based on CHAD S-2 score.

Plavix is NOT considered a superior choice in chronic A. fib.

➤ PHLEBOTOMY INDICATIONS IN CYANOTIC HEART DISEASE:

Hemoglobin **more than 22 Gm** <<<

Hematocrit **more than 65%** <<<

Hyperviscosity symptoms (**Headache, mental slowing**, etc.)

➤ SHOCK RESISTANT V FIB:

Treatment of choice: **AMIODARONE**

➤ NEW HYPERKALEMIA ON ACE/ARB/ALDACTONE THERAPY:

Switch to hydralazine/nitrate therapy.

This is shown as **the second best choice** to improve mortality in compared to placebo.

- **ANAPHYLACTIC REACTIONS:**
  - Can be **BIPHASIC**
  - **12 Hour Observation** is recommended to rule out later recurrence.

- **LINEZOLID THERAPY:**
  - Side Effects Include risk of Thrombocytopenia

- **ASPIRIN – SIDE EFFECTS:**
  - Can Cause **TINNITIS**
  - **Plavix dose NOT cause Tinnitis**

- **Selective Serotonin Re Uptake Inhibitors (SSRIs):**
  - Most SSRI can cause Anorgasmia and sexual dysfunction, except:
    - **BUPROPION** has LEAST risk of sexual Side Effects.
    - **MIRTAZAPINE**, has NO Sexual Side effects. It can cause WEIGHT Gain, so it is preferred in Anorexic patients.
    - **VENLAFAXINE** can raise Blood Pressure.

- **CIPROFLOXACIN – Drug Interaction:**
  - Can increase **Theophylline toxicity** by decreasing its clearance.

- **HYDRALAZINE - Side Effects:**
  - Hydralazine can cause Reflex Tachycardia
  - Avoid in Hypertensive patients with risk of Aortic Dissection

- **NON-COMPLICATED UTI (RECURRENT)**
  - OK for a Patient-initiated Antibiotic therapy plan, for non-complicated recurrent UTI.

- **HUMAN HERPES VIRUS INFECTIONS:**
  - **HHV 6+7:**
    - Hepatitis/Meningoencephalitis in immunocompromised patients.
  - **HHV 8:**
    - Kaposi Sarcoma

- **ACYCLOVIR resistant HERPES SIMPLEX viral infection:**
  - Switch to FOSCARNET. Risk of electrolyte imbalance
  - 2nd choice: CIDOFOVIR (but more NEPHROTOXIC)

- ## HERPES ZOSTER:
  - 1st Choice Rx: FAMCICLOVIR
  - Alt: VALACICLOVIR
  - STEROIDS: are OK to use for Zoster Pain, EXCEPT in patients with:
    - Uncontrolled DM,
    - Osteoporosis and
    - HTN
  - Prevention of Recurrence: ACYCLOVIR is effective, especially in Transplant Recepients

- ## CMV RETINITS IN HIV:
  - Sx: FLOATERS & BLURRED vision
  - 1st Line Rx: GANCICLOVIR: (only available as IV Rx)
  - 2nd Line Rx: **VAL**-GANCICLOVIR:
    - **Oral** form available.
    - Preferred for active lifestyle Pts.
    - Also for CMV prevention in TRANSPLANT patients.

- ## SECONDARY SYPHILIS:
  - **NO ORAL TREATMENT** REGIMENS
  - **IM BENZATHINE PENICILLIN** as **SINGLE-DOSE** is recommended for PRIMARY, SECONDARY, and EARLY-LATENT SYPHILIS.
  - 3 DOSES (ONCE WEEKLY) are recommended for LATE-LATENT SYPHILIS

- **MRSA SKIN infections:**
  - DOXYCYCLINE is appropriate empiric choice.
  - Other choices: Bactrim, Minocycline, Clindamycin
  - Levaquin and 1st Gen Cephalosporins do not cover MRSA

- **MRSA SPINAL OSTEOMYELITIS/DISK ABSCESS:**
  - **NO Neuro Deficits:**
    - Rx with **IV Antibiotics ONLY**
  - **WITH EVOLVING NEURO DEFICITS:**
    - URGENT DECOMPRESSION

- **Osteomyelitis in SICKLE CELL DISEASE Patients:**
  - Likely causative Organisms:
    - Staphylococcus
    - Streptococcus
    - **SALMONELLA** infection

- **CAT-BITE in PCN Allergic Patient:**
  - Rx with BACTRIM+CLINDAMYCIN.

- **LYME DISEASE (including CNS DISEASE) RX:**
  - CEFTRIAXONE (#1)
  - DOXYCYCLINE (#2)
  - PREVENTION after Tick-Bite:
    - SINGLE DOSE DOXYCYCLINE is highly effective for preventing Erythema Migrans after Tick bite (engorged, embedded tick on skin, found in endemic areas.

- **ISOLATION PROTOCOLS:**
  - PLAGUE (Pneumonic): DROPLET Precautions
  - Viral HEMORRHAGIC fever/SMALL POX:
    - AIRBORNE +CONTACT isolation.

- ## CHLAMYDIA SCREENING:
  - CDC Recommends Annual Screening for females <25 Years of age, with high risk status.
  - **AGE LESS THAN 25 YEARS** is the **STRONGEST risk** factor in the High Risk behavior population.

- ## HIV POST EXPOSURE PROPHYLAXIS:
  - If Source is HIV +: Start 2-3 Antiretroviral Drugs started for deep penetrating Injury. (PI + 2 NNRTI)?,

- ## ANTI-RETROVIRAL THERAPY (ART) CHOICES in HIV:
  - Based on
    - GENOTYPE RESISTANCE ASSAY
    - DETAILED DRUG HISTORY of prior ART use
  - Highly Active Anti-Retroviral Therapy **(HAART)**
    - Therapy Trigger: **CD4 Count <200** (regardless of symptom status)

- ➢ **HIV and PML (Progressive Multifocal Leukoencephalopathy)**
  - o **>>Start HAART ASAP**: 50% BETTER SURVIVAL
  - o PML: Multiple white matter lesions with mass effects

- ➢ **HIV and CNS LYMPHOMA**
  - o See with +ve EBV Serology
  - o Rx: RADIATION Therapy + STEROIDS

- ➢ **ANTI-TUBERCULOUS THERAPY (ATT):**
  - o Start with FOUR Drugs, if INH Resistance >4% in the Community.

- ➢ **CONTAMINATED LIPID SOLUTIONS**
    - o May contain MALASSEZIA FUR FUR organisms
    - o May induce systemic illness symptoms during IV infusions. Does not lead to Acute Cellulitis.

- ➢ **NECROTIZING FASCITIS (in IV Drug abuse Patients)**
    - o INITIAL Antibiotic Choice:
        - VANCO + ZOSYN + CLINDAMYCIN

- ➢ **Immunocompromised Patients with PCN Allergy:**
    - o AZTREONAM can be safely used.

- **Extended Spectrum Beta-Lactamase (ESBL) Gram Negative Rods (GNR)**
  - Rx of Choice: **CARBAPENEM (Aztreonam)**

- **C.Diff Colitis with PARALYTIC ILEUS:**
  - Rx: Start RECTAL VANCOMYCIN Administration

- **POST NEUROSURGERY PURULENT MENINGITIS:**
  - Empiric Therapy: Vancomycin + Cefipime

- ➤ **SUBDURAL EMPYEMA:**
  - ○ A Neurosurgical Emergency
  - ○ RX: Antibiotics + Neurosurgical **DRAINAGE**
  - ○ **Lumbar Puncture is Contraindicated**

- ➤ **Brain Abscess** with **Contiguous OTITIS** infection:
  - ○ RX: Ceftriaxone + Metronidazole

- ➤ **Neurosyphilis in Penicillin Allergic Patients:**
  - ○ **Proceed with PCN Desensitization as Penicillin is the only approved Rx option.**

- **Hepatitis A Vaccination:**
  - Administer 2 weeks before travel to high risk areas or other potential exposure risk.

- **Flu Vaccine :**
  - Avoid LIVE (nasal) flu shots in patients above 50 years of age, and those with chronic medical conditions, including heart Failure. Use inactivated injectable vaccine instead.

- **CRYPTOCOCCAL** infections in **Transplant** recipients:
  - Rx of Choice: **Flucytosine + Amphotericin** (Lipid Formulation)

- **Rx of PTSD (Post Traumatic Stress Disorder):**
  - **SERTRALINE** & **VENLAFAXINE** (FDA Approved choices)
  - Treat with medications and Psychotherapy.

- **Rx of PURULENT OTITIS EXTERNA :**
  - Physical Evacuation
  - Topical Antibiotics: Acetic Acid drops have local Antibiotic effects.
  - Topical Corticosteroids (reduce Inflammation)

- **COMMON WARTS TREATMENT:**
  - Salicylic Acid Prep (Topical) is preferred
  - 6-12 Week Treatment is needed.

- ## MIGRAINE THERAPY:
  - **TRIPTANS**: are **ABORTIVE** therapies. Less effective **DURING** and Attack.
  - **Metoclopramide** is effective during attack
  - Cutaneous Allodynia: Sensitive skin during Migraine attack.

- ## Upper Resp Tract Infection URI (Viral) Treatment:
  - Following therapies improve symptoms:
    - Pseudoephedrine
    - Atrovent Nasal Spray
    - Cromolyn Nasal inhaler
    - Humidified Air

- ## PSORIASIS: RX OPTIONS:
  - **Less than 5% of Body Surface Area**
    - High Dose corticosteroids Therapy x 2 weeks. May switch to other agents after 2 weeks.
    - **More than 5% Body Surface Area:**
      - PHOTOTHERAPY (1ST Line Rx for severe forms, i.e, Plaque and Guttate Psoriasis
      - Coal tar Solution
      - Methotrexate
    - **Facial Psoriasis:**
      - Tacrolimus Ointment

- **STATINS IN Acute Coronary Syndrome (ACS)**
  - **Start EARLY**, DEFINITELY before Hospital Discharge (provided no contraindications)

- **STATINS AND ANTIFUNGAL THERAPY:**
  - Itraconazole is contraindicated in patients taking statins.

- **TINEA VERSICOLOR: Rx**
  - Rx of choice; TOPICAL Ketoconazole, or TOPICAL Terbinafine (not Oral Preparations)

- **VARICELLA Vaccination for Healthcare Workers (HCW):**
    - All with negative Titer against Varicella
    - **LIVE VACCINE:**
        - OK to give to patients on less than 20 mg Prednisone Daily
        - VIRAL SHEDDING Occurs upto 4 weeks Post Injection
        - HCW to avoid contact with High Risk immunocompromised patients in the Hospital for FOUR WEEKS post vaccination.
        - Do Not give to Pregnant Patients.
        - Schedule: 2 doses 4-8 Weeks apart.

- **PANIC DISORDER - TREATMENT OPTIONS:**
    - **1st Line Rx: SSRI** (Selective Serotonin Reuptake Inhibitors), i.e, Paroxetine
        - Titrate Dose for Response
        - May add Low Dose benzodiazepines, for partial responders.
        - May also add Cognitive Behavioral therapy (CBT) as adjunct.
    - **2nd Line Rx: Atypical Neuroleptics:**
        - i.e, Resperidone, Olanzapine, Quetiapine

- **MINOR DEPRESSION:**
    - 1st Rx option:
        - Follow up Monitoring to asses stability and transitory symptom status, or progression to Organic Depression.

- **WEIGHT MANAGEMENT – DRUG THERAPY OPTIONS:**
    - **ORLISTAT:**
        - A Lipase Inhibitor, decreases Fat Absorption
        - May lose 2 – 2.5 Kg in 12 months time period.
    - **SIBUTRAMINE:**
        - Serotonin and Norepinephrine reuptake Inhibitor.
        - Suppresses Appetite
        - Avoid use in Uncontrolled Hypertension

- **Predictors of NPPV Failure:**
    - Resp Rate > 35
    - pH on Arterial Blood < 7.25
    - APACHE Score > 29
    - GCS Score < 11

- ➤ **ARDSNet Low Tidal Volume mechanical Ventilation in ARDS patients:**
  - o **Use Ideal Body Weight** to calculate target Tidal Volume.

- ➤ **Drug Induces Seizures:**
  - o Do not respond tp Phenytoin
  - o Rx Drug of choice: **Benzodiazepines**

- ➤ **HYDROGEN CYANIDE POISONING:**
  - o Unexplained **high Gap Lactic Acidosis**, not responsive to Oxygen and Fluid Resuscitation
  - o History **of combustion of Natural Fabrics** (wool, Silk etc.)
  - o RX: **Intravenous Sodium Thiosulphate**

- **Monitoring of Anticoagulation therapies**
  - **Factor X-a level Monitoring** can be used for monitoring **Heparin, LMWH, and Fondaparinux**. All of these act by catalyzing Anti Thrombin, which in turn deactivates Factor X-a.
  - **Factor X-a Monitoring cannot be used to monitor Argatroban or Leipirudin therapies as they are Direct thrombin Inhibitors.**

OPERATIVE AND PERI-OPERATIVE / TRANSPLANT CARE

➤ Criteria for MITRAL VALVE REPLACEMENT:

Symptomatic status: CHF, chest pain, LOC, etc.

Valve criteria:

    End-systolic dimension more than 45 mm

    End-diastolic dimension more than 60 mm

    EF less than 60%

➤ Repair of AORTIC ANEURYSM:

>>>Elective surgical repair criteria

    Male   **>5.5 cm**

    Female **4.5-5 cm**

>>> Refer for surgical evaluation for any rapidly changing aneurysm, i.e. >0.5 cm/year.

> ### PERIPHERAL VASCULAR DISEASE (PVD):

BETA BLOCKERS are indicated in the preoperative time period. Shown to reduce in-hospital and 30 day mortality in PVD patients.

> ### PARA-VALVULAR ABSCESS:

Echo **lucency**

"**URGENT** VALVE REPLACEMENT IS NEEDED"

> ### BRONCHIOLITIS OBLITRANS (BO)
> - A form of **chronic rejection post Lung transplant.**
> - **Early inspiratory Crackles** are characteristic.
> - **Severe airflow obstruction**

- **OBESITY:**
  - **NOT** associated with Higher risk of peri operative Pulmonary complication (>>BY ITSELF<<)

- **WHEEZING,** in an Asthmatic noted on **Pre-Op evaluation**:
  - Confers high risk for postoperative pulmonary complications.
  - RX: Optimize Asthma Treatment Plan.

- **PERI-OPERATIVE MEDICATIONS SCHEDULES:**
  - **DRUGS TO STOP ONE WEEK BEFORE SURGERY:**
    - SSRI
      - Increased risk of surgical bleeding
    - Estrogen Preparations and Estrogen Receptor Modulators (Tamoxifen):
      - Increased thromboembolism risk

  - **DRUGS that are OK TO CONTINUE:**
    - Nitrates, Beta Blockers, Statins and most Antihypertensives, except:
      - ACE-Inhibitors/ Angiotensin Receptor Blockers (ARB's) – can cause post op Hypotension – Hold AM doses on surgery day.
    - STATINS have anti-inflammatory plaque stability Effects. OK to continue till morning of Surgery.

- **TRAUMATIC AVULSION OF PERMANENT TEETH:**
  - Dental Care within 30 mins has the highest rates of successful reimplantation
  - Best transport medium for avulsed tooth:
    - #1: Put back in Socket
    - #2: Whole Milk

- **SURGICAL DVT Prophylaxis:**
  - **Elective Total Knee Replacement:**
    - High Dose LMWH: Enoxapain 30 mg SC Twice Daily
    - Alternate choice: Fondaparinux
    - Coumadin with target INR >2.5
    - Continuous Sequential Compression Devices (SCD)
  - **General Surgery DVT Prophylaxis:**
    - Low Dose LMWH: Enoxaparin 40 mg SC daily
    - Heparin 5000 Units SC BID/TID

WOMEN'S HEALTH

➢ VALVULAR HEART DISEASE IN PREGNANCY

Regurgitant valvular heart disease is **WELL TOLERATED** in pregnancy.

Functional status before pregnancy is a strong predictor of maternal risk.

➢ PREGNANCY AND HEART FAILURE

\>>> **RALES are NEVER NORMAL** in pregnancy

\>>> **AVOID ACE-Inhibitors** in pregnancy

\>>> Vasodilator Rx of choice in Pregnancy (Afterload reduction): **Hydralazine + Nitrates**.

➤ PREGNANCY AND ANTICOAGULATION GUIDELINES:

Warfarin: OK from SECOND TRIMESTER onwards.

LMWH/Heparin: OK with monitoring of factor X a level (LMWH), PTT(unfractionated heparin)

➤ PREGNANT FEMALES WITH MARFAN SYNDROME:

Increased risk of **AORTIC DISSECTION** during pregnancy

D/D of chest pain in pregnancy includes workup to rule out AORTIC DISSECTION.

➤ CHEST PAIN IN PREGNANCY:

Spontaneous coronary artery dissection can occur in pregnancy.

This can be confused with a myocardial infarction.

- **PREGNANT PATIENTS WITH UNREPAIRED EISENMENGER'S SYNDROME:**

  Carries **>50% risk of maternal mortality**

  Pregnancy is **strongly discouraged**

  VSD repair is not helpful after pulmonary hypertension is already established.

  Rx of choice: Heart lung transplant

  Afterload reduction contraindicated as it can decrease pulmonary blood flow and **can cause cardiovascular collapse**.

- **HOT FLASHES:**

  Alternative Therapies
  - Black Cohosh has been found to be helpful as treatment of Hot Flashes.

- **PREGNANCY AND HAART RX:**
  - OK to start HAART in 2nd Trimester, if indicated.
  - MAY start in 1st trimester for LATE STAGE HIV DISEASE (Low CD4 count and Thrush)
  - AVOID >> EFAVIRENZ (TERATOGENIC) <<
  - CAUTION: Check HEMOGLOBIN while Patients are on ZIDOVUDINE, as it can cause Anemia.

- **Pulmonary Embolism in Pregnancy:**
  - Treatment with Heparin or Low Molecular weight Heparin (LMWH) should be started
  - Continue for upto 6 weeks post-partum.

DIAGNOSTICS

➢ DOPPLER/ECHO SEVERITY CRITERIA FOR MITRAL VALVE REGURGITATION:

Regurgitant volume	>60 mL
Regurgitant fraction	>50%
Valve area	<0.4 cm²

➢ ONSET OF VENTRICULAR DYSFUNCTION IN VALVULAR HEART DISEASE

occurs when:

End-systolic LV dimension	>45 mm
LV Ejection fraction	<60%

➢ ANEMIA IN PATIENT WITH PROSTHETIC VALVE:

Suggests **risk of PARAVALVULAR ABSCESS**, (due to partial dehiscence or infection).

New onset CHF (within 6 months of valve replacement surgery) also raises the same concern.

> ## Test of choice for PFO, or cardiac source of emboli:

Transesophageal Echo (TEE) is the **BEST NONINVASIVE test** for the atrial septum evaluation.

HIGH RISK: Heparin (Low flow state, AFib, Previous clot Hx, Turbulent flow noted on echo.)

> ## CHOLESTEROL EMBOLI:

Increased risk after interventions.

May present as NEW ISCHEMIA after PCI procedure.

May NOT have limb mottling

+ urine eosinophilia

D/D: GOUT: Extremity is warm to touch in gout. + Increased **blood** eosinophil count.

> ## Diagnosis of PERICARDITIS:

<u>ST elevation and PR depression</u> is noted in MOST leads.

Pain is *<u>relieved by SITTING UP</u>*.

Pain <u>**radiates to the left shoulder**</u>.

➤ Diagnosis of CARDIAC AMYLOIDOSIS:

LOW VOLTAGE on EKG

But, THICK MYOCARDIAL WALL on echo. *(discordance)*

DIAGNOSIS: Abdominal fat pad biopsy.

➤ BUNDLE BRANCH BLOCK ON EKG:

RBBB = "**Rabbit ears**" in **V1**

LBBB = exaggerated LVH changes with **wide QRS in V6**.

➤ RANSON'S CRITERIA:
Since 1974

A score of more than 8 shows significant risk of Pancreatic Necrosis

Criteria on Admission: (GA-LAW)

- **G**lucose more than 200 mg/dL
- **A**ge more than 55 Years
- **L**DH more than 35
- **A**ST more than 250
- **W**BC more than 16K
-

Criteria at 48 Hours: (CHOBBS)

- **C**alcium Level Less than 8 gm
- **H**ematocrit fall more than 10%
- **O**xygen (PaO2) less than 60
- **B**UN increase by 5+
- **B**ase Deficit More than 4 meq/L
- **S**equestration of Fluid, more than 6L

➢ CENTOR Criteria for GABHS

(Group A Beta Hemolytic Streptococcal Infection): Assigns One Point each for,
- Fever
- Tonsillar Exudates
- Cervical Lymphadenopathy
- Cough

➢ BIRADS (Breast Imaging Reporting and Data Systems)
- BENIGN: Category 1,2,3
- SUSPCIOUS for Malignancy: Category 4
- Highly Suggestive of Malignancy: Category 5

➢ OBESITY CLASSIFICATION:
- WHO STANDARD DEFINES OBESITY AS BMI >30
- CLASS I: 30 – 34.9
- CLASS II : 35 – 39.9
- CLASS III: >40

- ➤ **"HALO" SIGN on Chest X-Ray:**
    - ○ Nodule in center with Ground-glass changes around it : suggests **ASPERGILLUS** infection.

- ➤ **CHYLOTHORAX:**
    - ○ **HIGH Triglycerides > 110 mg/dl**
    - ○ **LOW Cholestrol** Concentration
    - ○ **d/d: Pseudo-Chylothorax:** Cholestrol is >200 mg/dl in pseudochylothorax, with cholesterol crystals on light microscopy.

- ➤ **"RING ENHANCING"** Lesions on **CT Head**:
    - ○ Rule out **NOCARDIAL INFECTION**
    - ○ **Modified AFB Stain** is POSITIVE
    - ○ Rx: **BACTRIM**
    - ○ Risk Factors:
        - ▪ Immunocompromised status
        - ▪ CHRONIC Steroid therapy

- **20-30-40 Rule:**
  - Used to decide **need for intubation** in neuromuscular disease patients with respiratory Failure.
    - Vital Capacity < 20 ml/Kg
    - Max Insp Pressure (MIP) < 30 cm H2O
    - Max Exp Pressure (MEP) < 40 cm H2O
    - & inability to maintain secretions

- **OTTAWA RULE:**
  - To Assess need for Ankle Films
    - Only when tenderness noted at:
      - Posterior edges of Medial/Lateral malleolus
      - Navicular Bone medially
      - Base of 5th Metatarsal Laterally

- ➢ **PPD PARAMETERS:**
    - ○ HEALTHY Adults + NO EXPOSURE = >15 MM
    - ○ ABNORMAL X-ray (APICAL DISEASE) = >5 MM
    - ○ HIV, TRANSPLANT Patients = >5MM
    - ○ HIGH RISK = >10mm

    (Healthcare workers; Prisoners; Immigrants > 5yr; Patients with cancer, Diabetes, IVDA, Renal failure, recent weight loss)

- ➢ **EOSINOPHILS IN CSF on Lumbar Puncture**
    - ○ Eosinophilic Meningitis
    - ○ Caused by: "**Rat-Lung Worm**": AKA *Angiostrongylus Cantonensis*: (Most common cause worldwide)
    - ○ Risk Factors:
        - **Uncooked SNAILS**, and
        - Contaminated vegetables

- ➢ **HERPES SIMPLEX ENCEPHALITIS (HSV)**
    - ○ Preferred Diagnostic Test
        - PCR of CSF
        - >90% sensitivity & Specificity

- ➤ **FOOT ULCER with risk for OSTEOMYELITIS:**
    - Recommend BONE BIOPSY and Histopathology Examination BEFORE starting Antibiotics.

- ➤ **HIV: LAB Diagnosis:**
    - **WESTERN BLOT is Gold standard** for HIV Diagnosis
    - HIV RNA Viral load can be a misleading test
    - **ELISA +ve / Western Blot –ve** : Cross Reactive Antibodies (HIV NEGATIVE)
    - **ELISA +ve / Western Blot +ve** : HIV POSITIVE (or SEROCONVERSION)

- ➤ **CLUE CELLS:**
    - Diagnostic for BACTERIAL VAGINOSIS
    - Gram Negative Rods Attached to Vaginal Epithelial cells
    - D/D: Vaginal Candidiasis: Budding Yeast on examination.

- ➢ **HEPATITIS C :**
  - o Diagnostic Test of Choice:
    - ▪ **Qualitative HCV RNA Viral load** is the **MOST SENSITIVE** Diagnostic test available.

- ➢ **CARDIAC ARRYTHMIAS - DETECTION:**
  - o Continuous 30-Day Event Loop Recorder is preferred if inpatient observation, telemonitoring and cardiac workup is non-diagnostic.
  - o Loop recording study is Preferred over the EP Study.

- ➢ **Abdominal Aortic Aneurysm (AAA) Screening:**
  - o Recommended for Patients **65-75 years of Age**, who **EVER SMOKED**.

- **DIAGNOSIS OF BONE METASTASES:**
  - **BONE SCAN** is the BEST Diagnostic test for bone mets as it picks up "HOT SPOTS", related to **OSTEOBLASTIC** activity.
  - **PET Scan is not preferred** as it picks up OSTEOCLASTIC foci better.

INTERPRETATIONS SKILLS

➢ ANKLE - BRACHIAL INDEX (ABI):

Normal: LE pressure **>** U E pressure

(Normal value = **11.3**)

    <0.4 = SEVERE ARTERIAL OBSTRUCTION

    > 1.3 = CALCIFIED vessels (noncompressible)

    0.4 - 0.9 = MODERATE arterial obstruction.

➢ TIMI SCORE:

Used for **Risk stratification** in ST elevation MI.

Based on **Age, Medical history, Physical exam, and Presentation**.

Range = 0-14.

0-2/low risk

3-4/intermediate risk

5-7/high risk. >>> *Early invasive approach recommended for her high-risk status based on TIMI score.*

- ➤ **CURB-65:**
  - For COMMUNITY ACQUIRED PNEUMONIA:
  - Level of care Planning score:
  - <u>C</u>onfusion, <u>U</u>rine output, <u>R</u>esp rate, <u>B</u>UN, Age><u>65</u> Yrs.

- ➤ **AORTIC DISSECTION – CLASSIFICATION Systems:**
  - **STANFORD Type A:**
    - **DeBakey-I:** From Ascending Aorta onwards till Abdomen.
    - **DeBakey – II:** Starts and Stops at Ascending Aorta
  - **STANFORD Type B:**
    - **DeBakey – III:** Starts at Descending Aorta.

About this Book:

SALIENT FEATURES:

- Quick LAST MINUTE review ideal for:
    - USMLE Step-III candidates
    - Anyone needing to update themselves with the latest advances in Practical General Internal Medicine within the shortest possible time, including:
        - Medical Residents, Post Graduate Fellows, Nurse Practitioners, Physician Assistants,
        - Family Practice and Primary Care Physicians,
        - Specialist candidates (in specialties other than Internal medicine) taking Qualifying Medical Examinations,
- Unique "Flash Bullet" format ideal for quick memorization, and recall, as and when needed.
- Focused "No- Frills Abstract" content to aid visual retention of important facts, in shortest possible timeframe.

www.ingramcontent.com/pod-product-compliance
Lightning Source LLC
Chambersburg PA
CBHW041100180526
45172CB00001B/41